WHY RAW VEGAN?

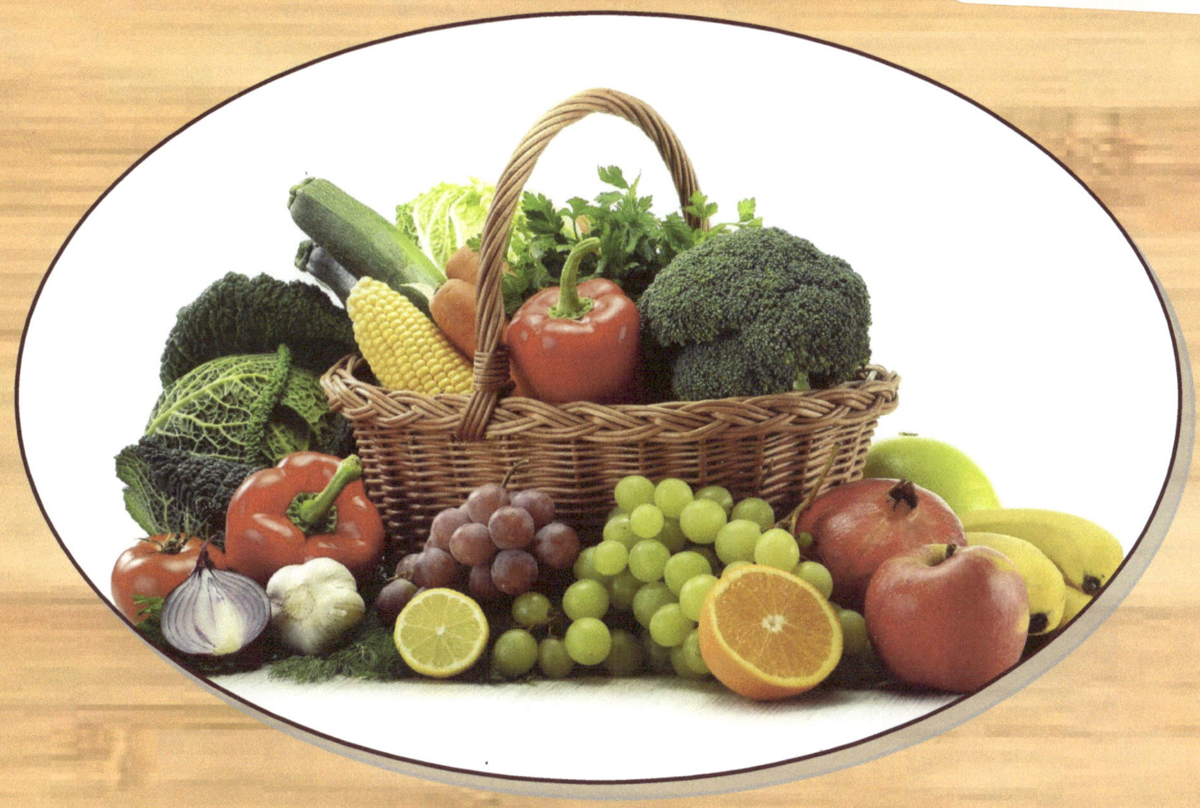

by

Alice Dee

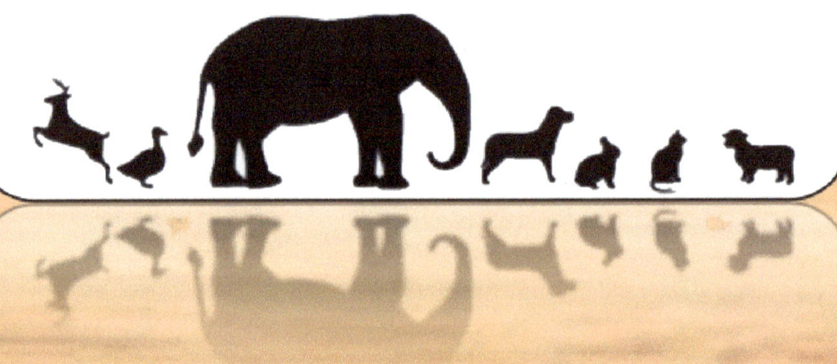

The greatness of a nation and its
moral progress can be judged
by the way its animals are treated.
- Gandhi

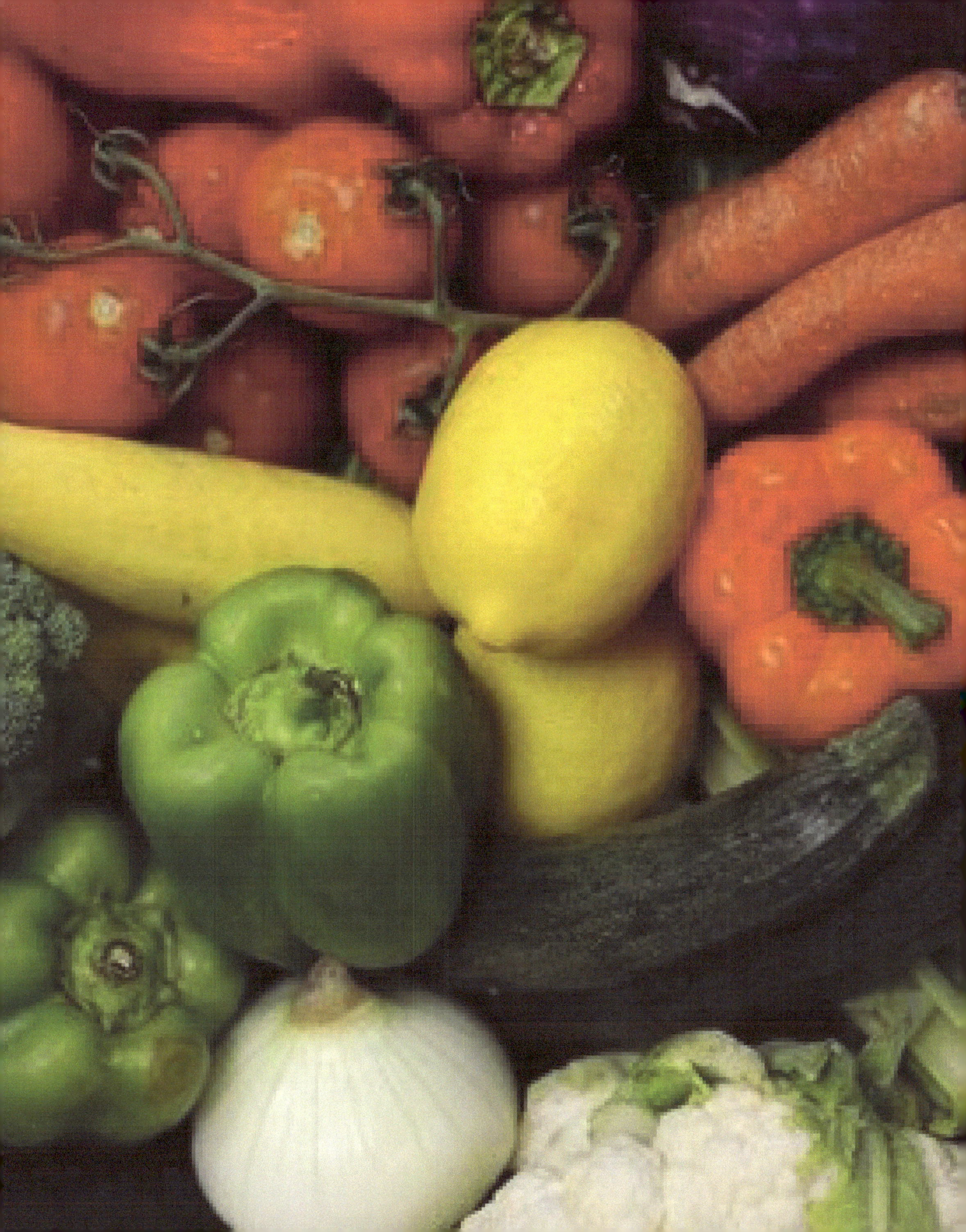

TABLE OF CONTENTS

Meat is Just Unnecessary

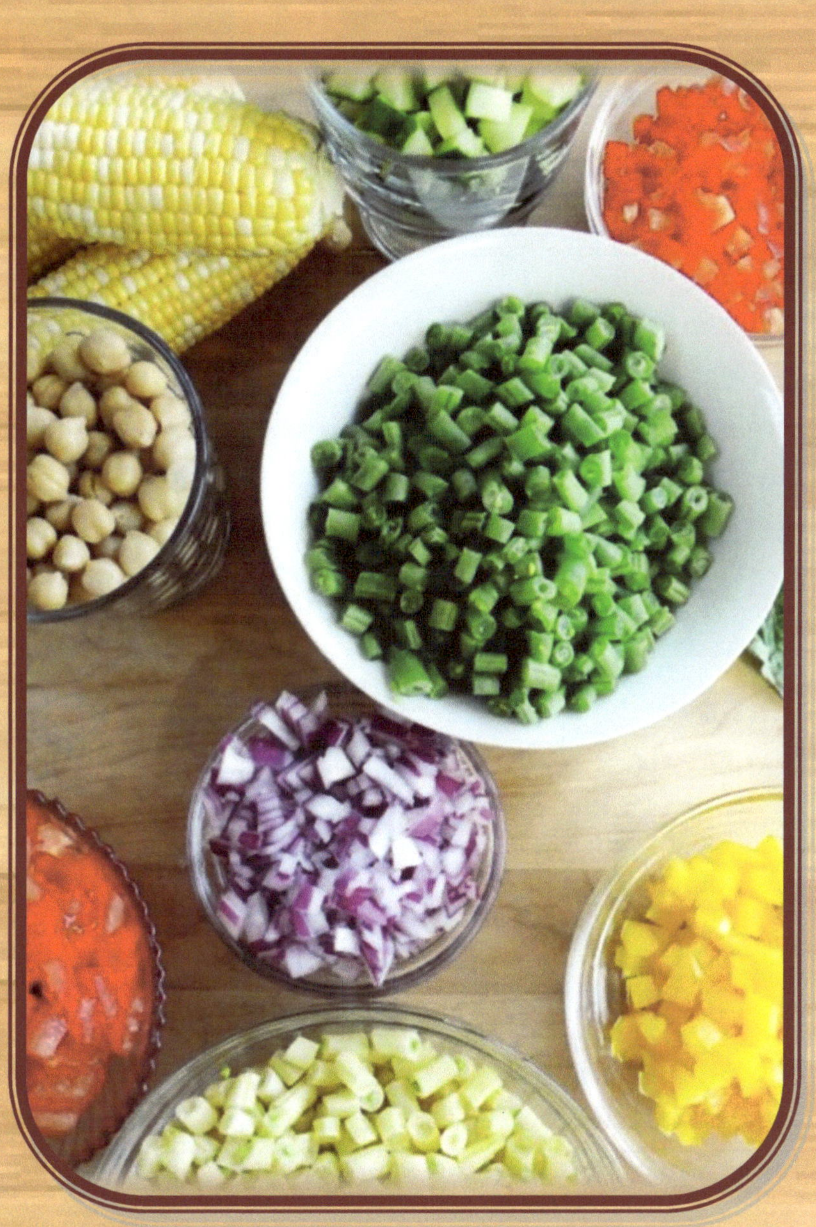

First of all, everyone needs to understand that no matter what you might have thought, read or been taught, meat and other animal products are unnecessary, unnatural, unkind and even unhealthy for humans.

These facts have been known for thousands of years in the East where most Buddhists, Jains and many Hindus refrain from eating meat for their entire lives on compassionate grounds. At the present time, there exist an estimated 150 million vegan humans and around 350 million vegetarian humans on the planet, who can also personally vouch for the fact that flesh foods are completely unnecessary for humans.

Furthermore, the production of meat and other animal products is very wasteful of human-edible food and causes food shortages for humans. Instead of feeding many times the amount of plant food humans can eat to animals in order to eat their flesh, we can instead be feeding it to humans directly.

The production of meat is also very damaging to the environment. It is presently the leading cause of deforestation on the planet, and manure pools from intensive animal agricultural facilities have polluted waterways and oceans, causing loss of life and serious ecological damage. In addition, animal agriculture is presently the primary single cause of climate change, and the methane produced by overpopulated farmed animals, and especially cows, is 84 times more potent than carbon dioxide due to its effectiveness in absorbing heat.

Last, but certainly not least, meat production causes great suffering and an untimely death for the sentient creatures it is violently obtained from. Fortunately, you can keep your conscience entirely clear of such cruelty by eating a vegan diet.

Be Like the Raw Vegan Gorilla

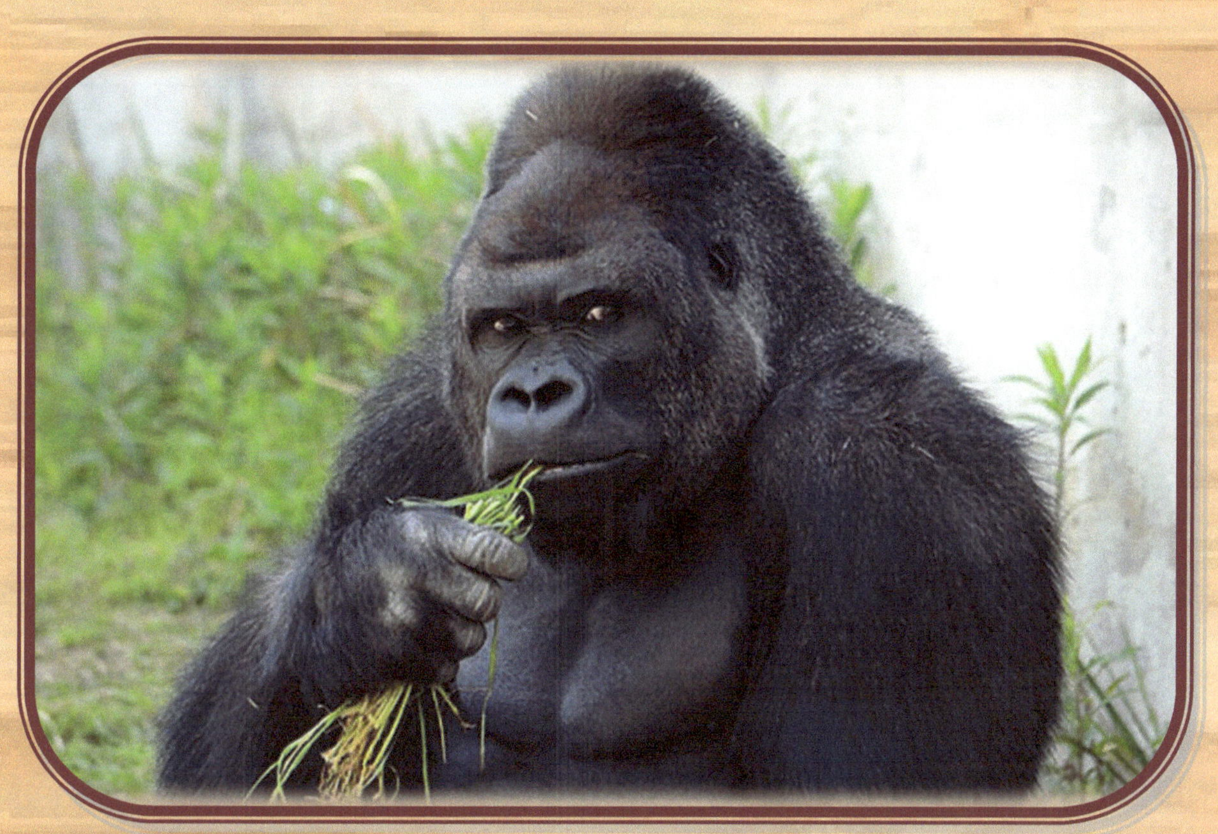

Meat and other animal products are not a significant part of the natural diet of any great ape, like our very muscular close cousins the mighty gorillas who are overwhelmingly vegan after weaning and only eat raw food.

Chimpanzees and orangutans also consume a largely plant-based diet focused on fruits, nuts and green plants. Like the gorilla, they sometimes also eat a modest amount of social insects like termites, which human vegans usually replace in their diets with legumes and/or nuts and a vitamin tablet containing miniscule amounts of Vitamin B12.

While the babies of other great apes do consume milk produced by their mothers, beyond the age of weaning, they do not do so. They also do not consume milk produced by another species, which often has a very different nutritional profile that depends on the species it came from.

Like the other great apes, humans are not properly adapted to consume meat from a physiological standpoint, and it even often make them chronically ill when they consume it. In contrast to true carnivores whose physiology has been specifically adapted to consuming flesh foods, humans are perfectly able to subsist very healthily on a fully raw and plant-based diet once weaned from their mothers' milk.

Basically, if mature gorillas, chimps and orangutans do not need meat, cow milk, cheese or other animal products to subsist on as part of their natural diets — and do not need to cook their plant foods either — then neither do humans.

Choose the Apple
Not the Rabbit

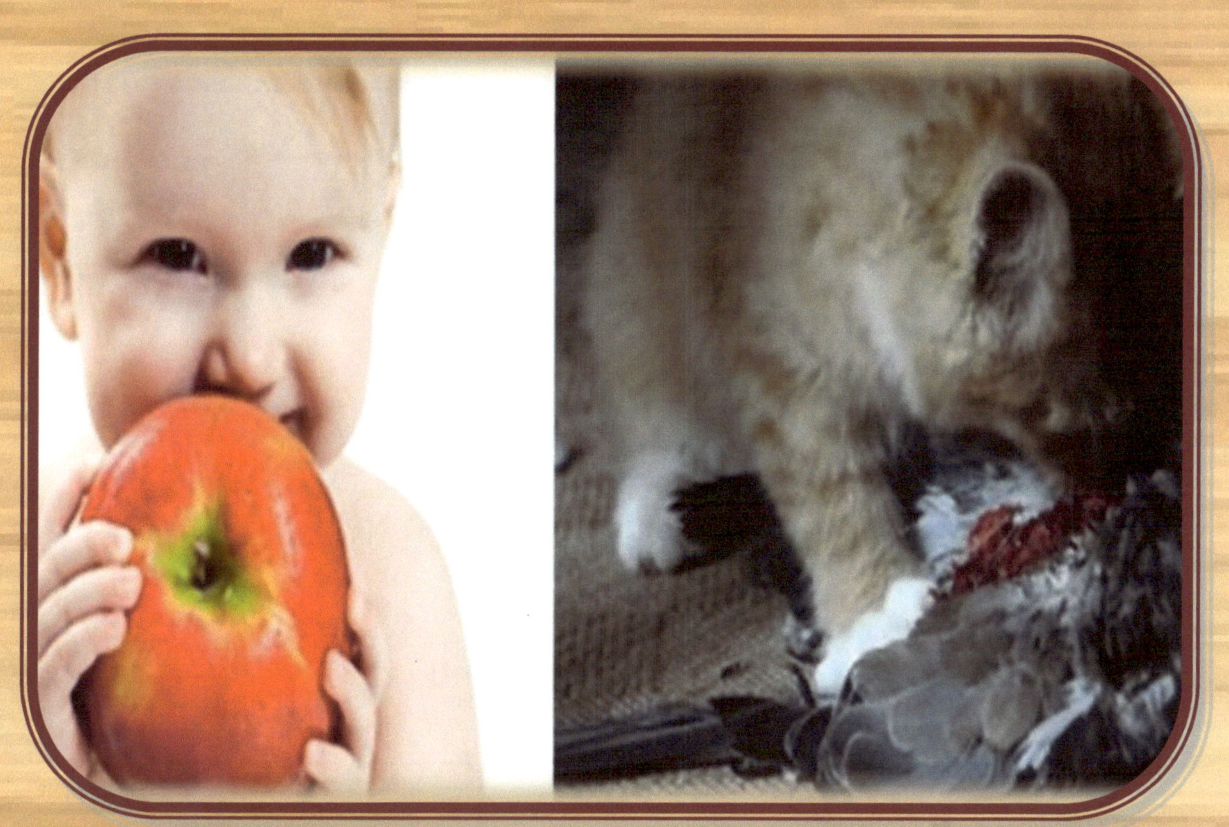

Unfortunately, eating meat also involves killing, which most humans find instinctively and ethically repulsive since they would not wish to be killed themselves. This is a simple application of the ethical gold standard of reciprocity, sometimes called the Golden Rule, which says that you should not do to others what you would not wish to be done to you.

To understand that killing is not instinctive or normal for humans, consider for a moment the choice of a human baby between munching on a nice ripe apple versus killing and eating a friendly bunny rabbit. The baby will virtually always instinctively do the compassionate and decent thing and choose to eat the apple and play with the rabbit. That behavior is what comes naturally to humans. Contrast that with a predator's instinct to kill to eat, such as what a cat might do to a bird.

It is only later in life that many humans are taught — and sometimes even forced — to eat flesh and even to hunt and kill their fellow creatures who do not want to die, when such acts not only offend their conscience but can also damage their long term health and reduce their lifespan when they consume flesh foods and other animal products high in saturated fats.

Furthermore, humans lack the physiological means to kill animals and rip apart their bodies with the equipment they were naturally endowed with. They have no sharp teeth or claws, they do not run very fast, they have a weak sense of smell for tracking, and they are not very strong. They also cannot safely consume raw meat. They are therefore largely unable to catch, kill, butcher and eat other creatures without unnatural things like weapons, knives and fire. Like gorillas, humans are instead well -adapted to eating raw plant foods, just as raw vegans do.

Avoid Killing
Food by Cooking It

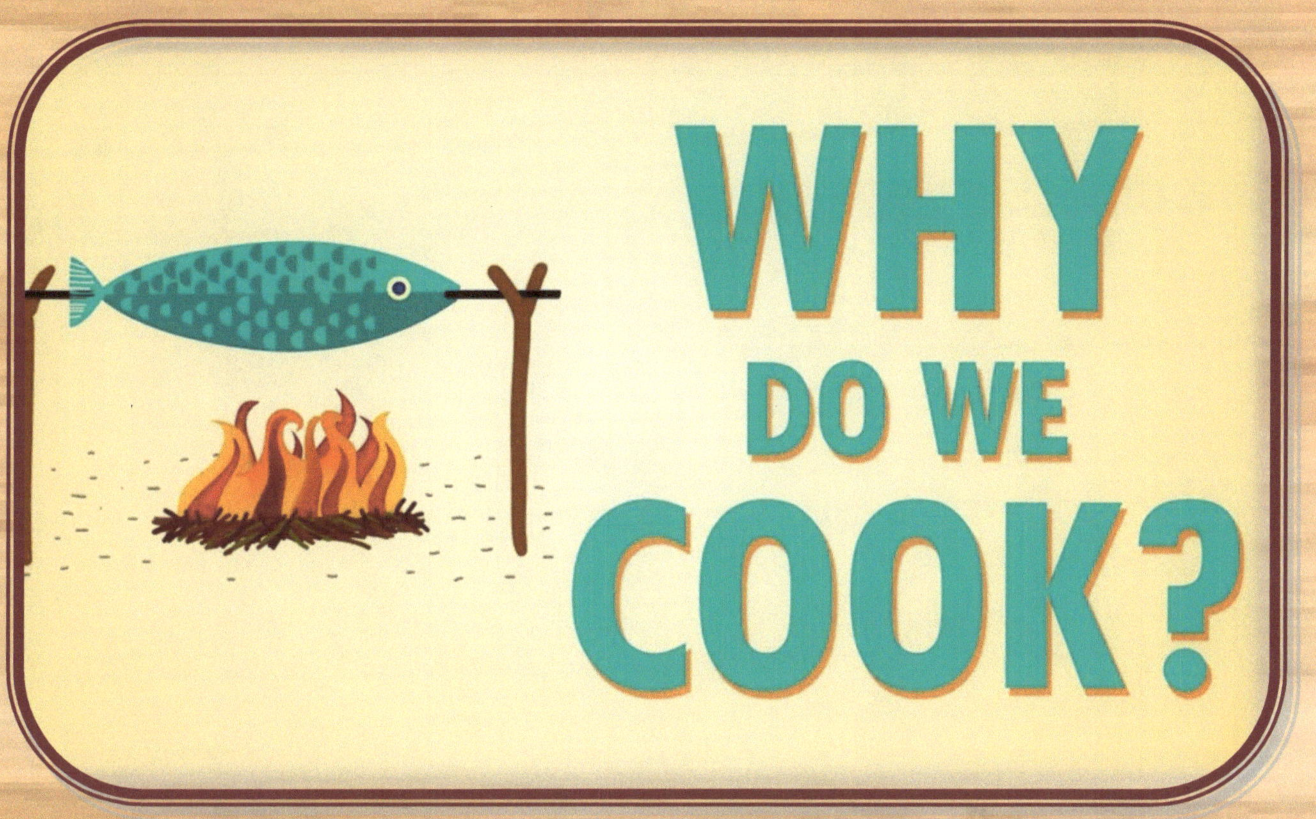

WHY
DO WE
COOK?

Basically, humans are the only animals who kill their food by cooking it above the temperature of the sun on a hot day, which is about 117 degrees Fahrenheit. Not only does this unnatural process eliminate vital nutrients and precious biophotons from foods, but cooking also denatures digestive enzymes contained in food when it is heated above 117 degrees F. This damage done by excessive heat causes us to waste substantial amounts of energy to create these enzymes ourselves in order to digest cooked food.

Unlike any other living creature, humans seem to have evolved this rather peculiar habit of cooking their food relatively recently in their history and probably because it generally makes them sick to eat raw meat that would not ordinarily be a natural part of their diet. Of course, this does not mean humans need to persist in destroying nutrients, biophotons and enzymes in the healthful raw plant foods they were properly adapted to consume.

Humans might also cook food seeking to kill unseen "germs" in food by cooking it. Still, despite being greatly feared by many humans and the subject of intensive product marketing campaigns to remove them, such tiny creatures actually seem to have very little to do with causing illness in a human. The presence of infectious agents actually seem to be more of a symptom instead, as will be discussed further in the next section.

Furthermore, those people whose immune systems are properly strengthened and nourished by consuming a natural diet consisting of nutritious, whole and fully raw plant foods typically have very little to fear from consuming the vast majority of plant foods without cooking them.

Fight Germs with Good Gut Flora

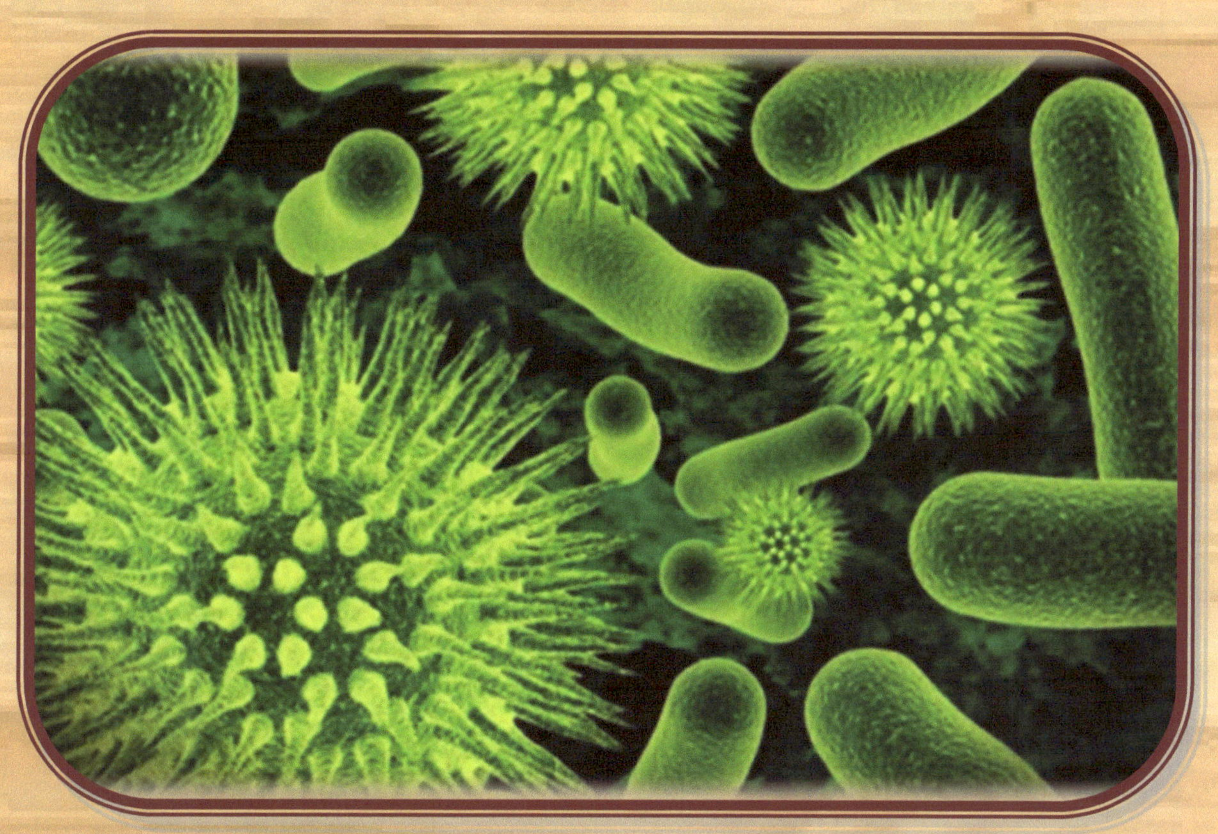

Studies show that consuming a vegan diet considerably strengthens the colony of friendly bacteria residing in your digestive system, also known as beneficial gut flora, that helps you fight and resist unfriendly germs. Those humans who consume flesh foods typically harbor greater amounts of less friendly organisms that can also harm their health.

While some people resort to cooking their food in an attempt to eliminate "germs", having healthy vegan gut flora generally does the job much better. Consuming plant foods raw not only does not destroy the valuable vitamins and other heat-sensitive micronutrients in the food you eat that cooking does, but it also allows friendly probiotics to enter your body.

By cooking food, humans also consistently weaken their immune systems by not exposing them to a broader variety of stimuli in modest doses for them to develop immunity against. In addition, they thoroughly denature all of the proteins and enzymes contained in food by cooking it, thereby making proper digestion so much more difficult and energy-consuming that contributes to the accelerated aging process and chronic low energy levels that flesh, dairy and egg-eaters usually experience.

Cooking also softens dietary fiber and thereby weakens its gut-cleansing effect that has many health benefits and significantly improves digestive throughput, which also helps remove dietary toxins promptly. When consumed raw, such dietary fiber also prevents a myriad of digestive diseases — including bowel cancer — largely by reducing and removing toxic accumulations in the digestive system.

Stay Young with an Alkaline Body pH

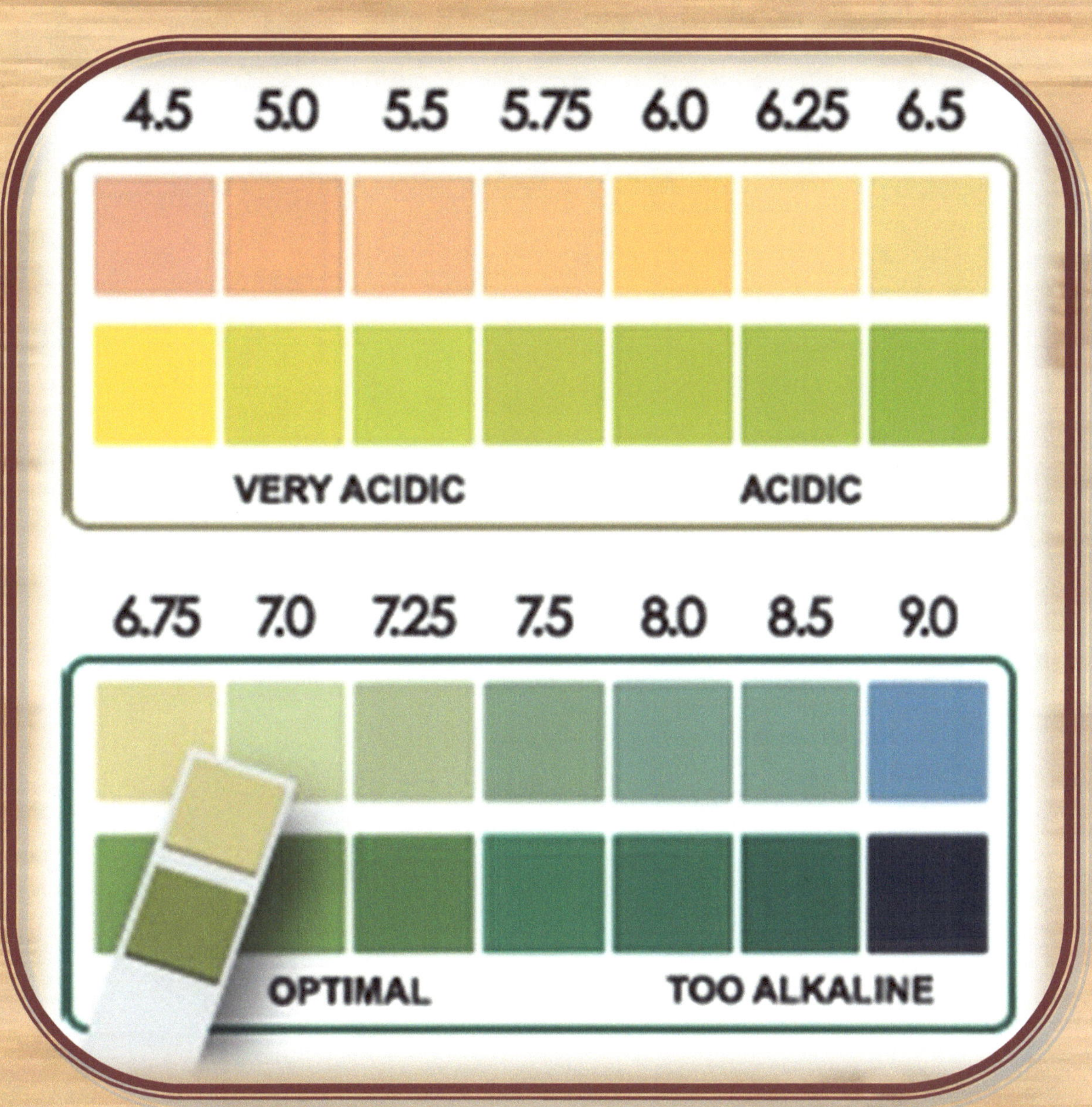

Performing the clearly unnatural act of consuming cooked food also ultimately has an acidifying effect on the pH of our bodies, since all cooked food promotes the formation of body acidity. Furthermore, certain cooked foods — especially animal products like meat, eggs and dairy — promote even more acid formation than others in the human body and can therefore cause substantial harm to our health.

Among other things, this acidity causes mucus accumulation, cellular breakdown and various forms of disease, in contrast to the healthful rejuvenating effect that consuming alkalizing raw foods generally has on the human body. These adverse effects are particularly notable with milk, which has become difficult — and even illegal in some places — to get in its raw form these days unless you get it from a human mother or keep dairy animals and milk them yourself.

Another amazing and related benefit of the raw vegan diet is that long term fully raw vegans tend to regain and keep a remarkable appearance of youthfulness. Since raw vegans typically have a more alkaline body pH due to their alkalizing plant-based diet — and they also expend far less energy in digestion by keeping their food's enzymes active — they tend to age at a slower rate overall. Numerous examples exist of long term raw vegans looking 10-20 years younger than their biological age.

Part of the reason for this observed youthfulness of raw vegans is that maintaining unhealthy over-acidic pH levels in your body can lead to the early breakdown of tissues and hence premature aging. So the good news is that you can both stay healthy and look younger as a raw vegan!

The Raw Food Pyramid

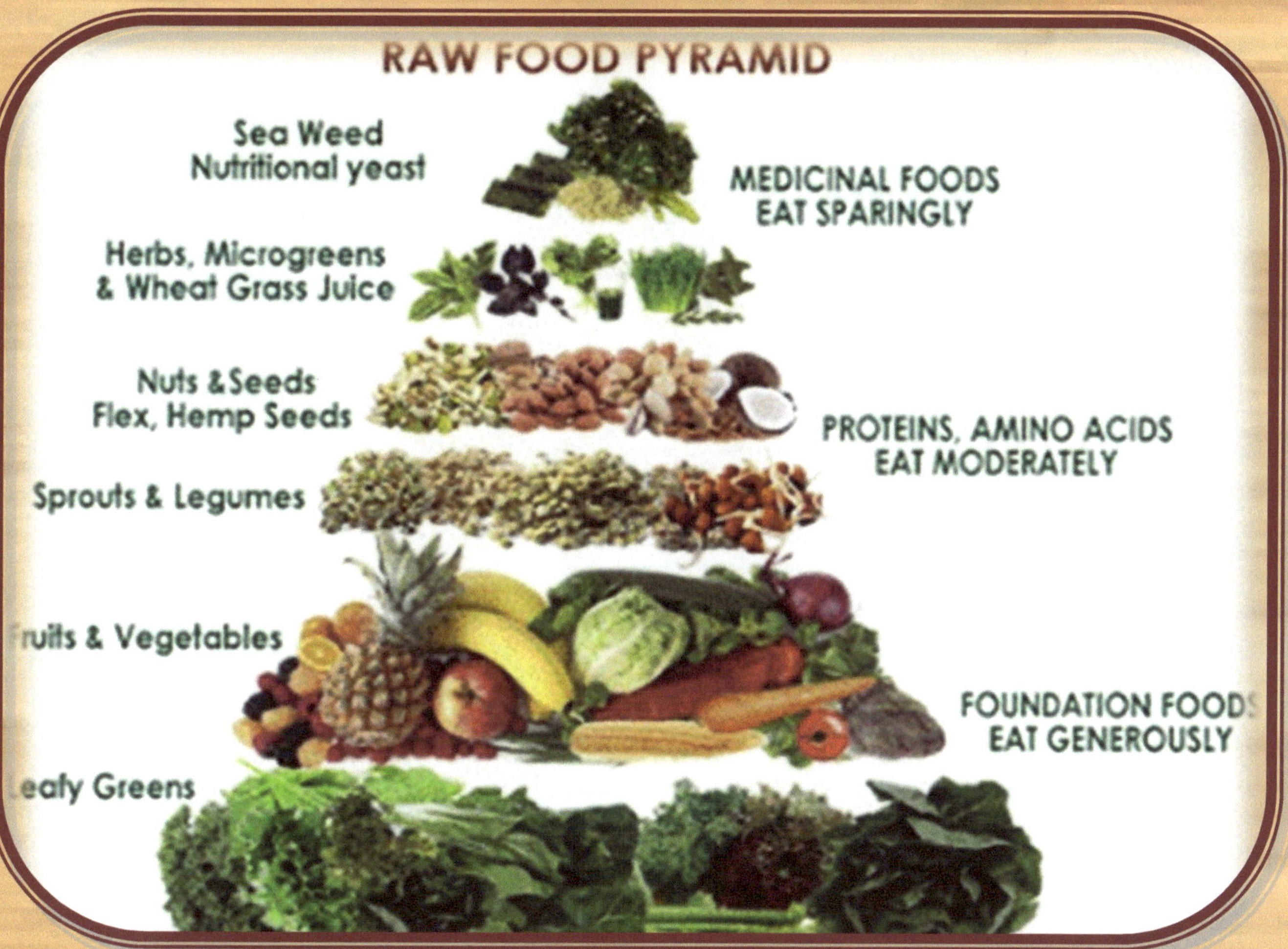

The type of food raw vegans should be consuming and the approximate amounts of each food type are shown in the raw food pyramid depicted on the opposing page. The general categories consist of the following:

(1) **Foundation Foods** - At the bottom of the pyramid are foods like leafy greens that raw vegans can eat in abundance. Above the greens are most of the other fruits and vegetables. They have lots of fiber and healthful nutrients.

(2) **Protein Foods** - These foods should be eaten moderately by raw vegans. They start with sprouted legumes and grains like chick peas, mung beans, lentils, wheat and rye. On the higher rung are nuts, seeds and coconut meat.

(3) **Medicinal Foods** - These foods should be eaten sparingly by raw vegans. The lower part of this tier starts with things like herbs, microgreens, wheatgrass juice and spirulina, while the highest tier of the pyramid includes foods like seaweed. The image also mentions nutritional yeast, which is not generally a raw food, but it does contain helpful nutrients for vegans — like Vitamin B12 and other B complex vitamins in most cases — so it is often used to impart a cheesy flavor and extra micronutrients to vegan foods.

To obtain my favorable results with the raw vegan diet, I followed this general pyramid pattern when eating and stuck strictly to the diet at around 95% organic and 100% raw. I found it easier to do this with the help of my raw vegan restaurant while it was operating.

My own experience with the diet was that it was exceptionally rejuvenating and energizing, as well as being excellent for weight loss and creating a positive mental attitude. Since my diet was also somewhat experimental at the time, I also hoped to make a positive example of myself for others to consider following since the raw vegan diet seemed to be working out so well for me.

Enjoy Effective
Weight Loss

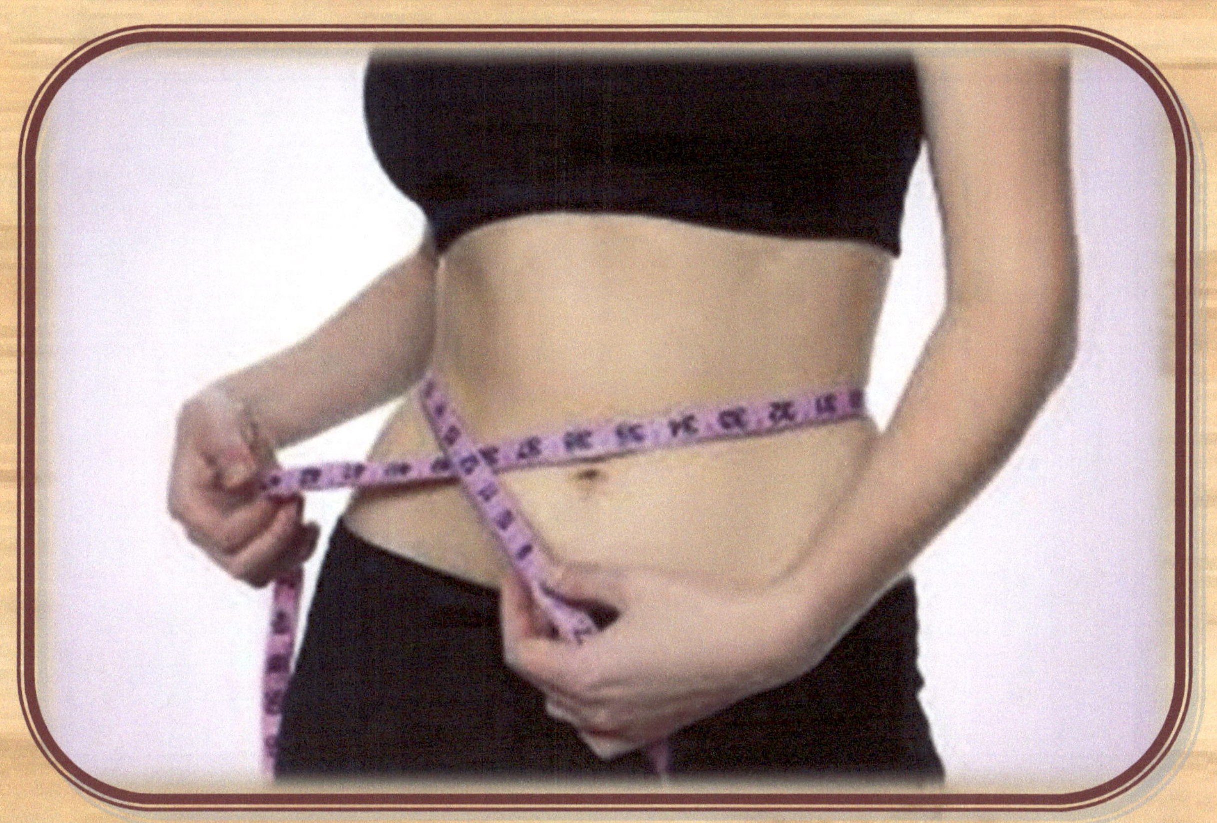

A particularly welcome result of the raw vegan diet I followed was its notable slimming effect. After following the fully raw vegan diet for several months, I discovered that I had lost 40 stubborn pounds that I had gained while recently pregnant.

I eventually slimmed down to weigh as little as 110 pounds in just a few months, which was quite amazing for my tall and medium-built body frame. I even became a little concerned about the weight loss continuing any further, but my weight stabilized there as I started to add more calorie-dense foods containing healthful fats to my diet like nuts, seeds and avocados. Also, I felt just great!

My body shape also transformed as my stomach flattened and my flabby belly pouch completely disappeared, along with all of the unsightly cellulite that had accumulated over the years on my hips and thighs. I felt renewed!

Many other people have also discovered the remarkable slimming effects of a raw vegan diet that all other animals eating a raw diet already benefit from. Think about it, have you ever seen an overweight deer living wild? Probably not since they eat only the raw foods they are adapted to eat.

In fact, if you start from a moderate weight, it is actually quite a challenge to carry any excess weight after several months on a raw vegan diet. As that weight melts off, you will feel free of the excess burden on your joints and energy levels that it imposes. For me, it was like having a large 40 pound backpack taken off me, and I felt freer, lighter and much more agile! I also felt more comfortable exercising around other people and felt better about myself in general.

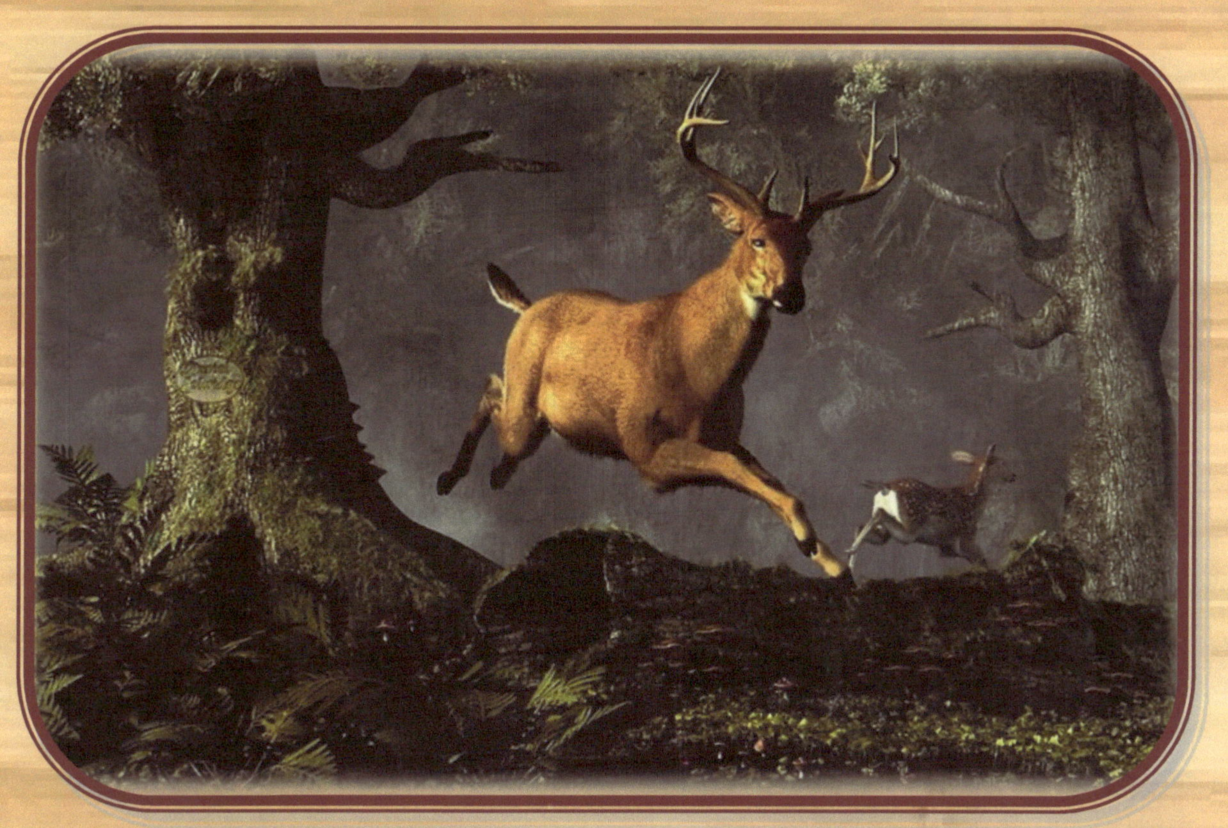

Maintaining the raw vegan diet consistently also provided me with plenty of energy over the years I followed it. I not only felt clearer on a mental and spiritual level, but I also found that I could work, exercise and hike with great stamina. In fact, I felt a lot like I expect a bounding deer running through the woods might feel when I was out hiking!

As another welcome side effect of the fully raw vegan diet, I became exceedingly happy to the point of even being quite blissful at times, although I was also able to focus, meditate and work whenever necessary. In addition, I generally enjoyed perfect health and digestion, with no colds, flu, mucus accumulation or any other signs of illness after my brief Herxheimer or detox reaction cleared up. Also called a die-off reaction, this event that some people starting a raw vegan diet experience to a greater or lesser extent felt a bit like the flu to me.

Fortunately, I was informed in advance by my experienced friends that this reaction is a perfectly normal initial result of following this healing diet. It takes place as bacteria and/or yeast die off and release toxins when you no longer feed them with unhealthy and unnatural food for your species.

If you do experience something similar in the early days of following a fully raw vegan diet, you can probably just persist and it will very likely clear up after about a week, depending on how much detoxification your body requires. Your energy levels should then improve greatly. If it goes on for longer than that, you might like to consult with your doctor to make sure you are progressing well.

Let Food be Your Medicine

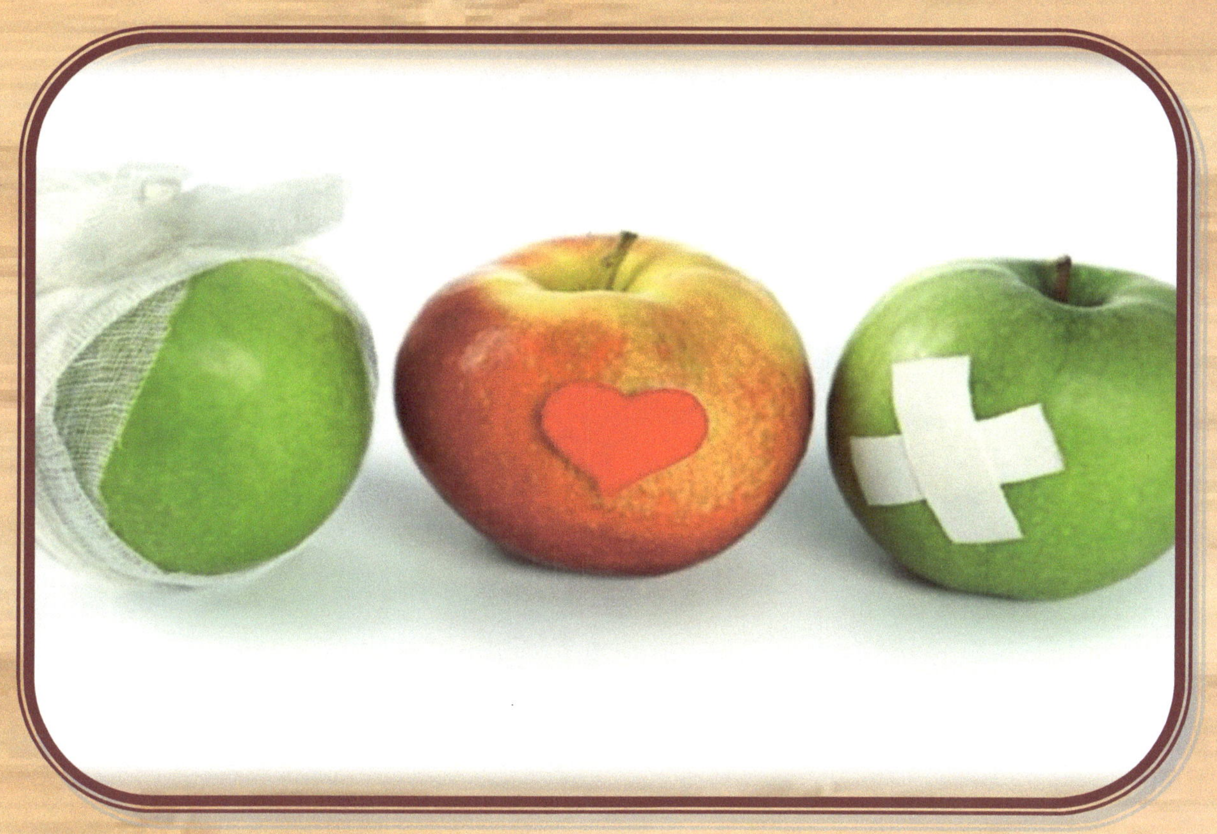

I found the raw vegan diet very healing, and I felt in excellent physical and mental health overall while on the diet after my initial detox reaction cleared up quickly. In fact, it was the best I can ever recall feeling in my entire life.

Some of my friends did probably think I was a bit thin for a while and maybe even a bit too happy, but that only left me wondering if perhaps they were just a bit jealous of my remarkable physical, mental and spiritual transformation the raw vegan diet facilitated.

As far as dietary healing is concerned, I would strongly recommend using the vegan raw food diet for treating health conditions such as obesity, Type II diabetes, some cancers and skin disorders, high blood cholesterol levels and arterial clogging problems. Since those are serious health issues, using the raw vegan diet as a treatment plan under the supervision of a health professional would be strongly advisable. For diabetics, I am aware of inpatient clinics that specialize in supervising patients while undergoing treatment with the raw vegan diet for that condition with good success.

The raw vegan diet also helps improve certain types of digestive problems, especially those involving enzyme deficiencies or constipation. Also, people with complexion issues like severe acne often find they clear up remarkably well while on a raw vegan diet.

The diet is also a great energizing, detoxification and rejuvenation diet to either maintain long term or to periodically use as needed to counteract the adverse effects of aging, stress and environmental toxins on the body.

Eat Raw From The Garden

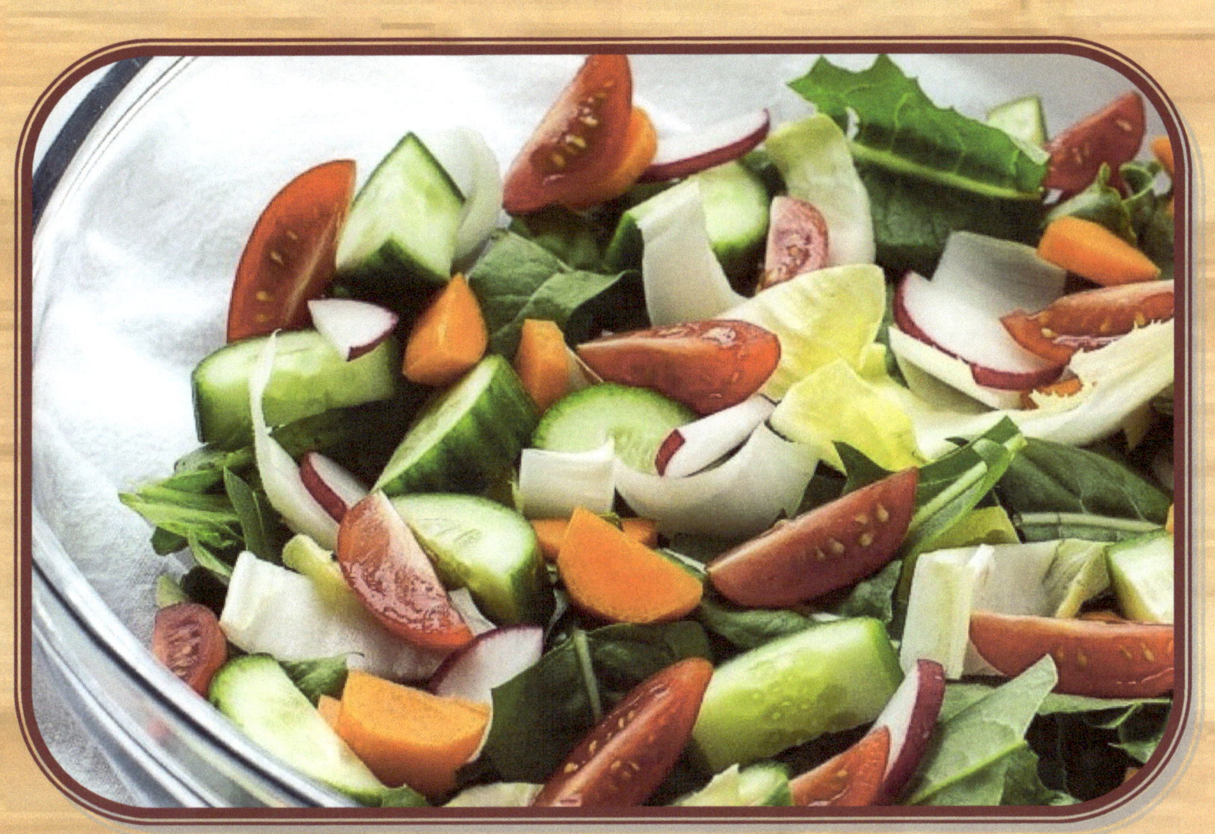

Raw vegans typically aim to get back to their gardens by consuming a whole food plant-based diet for that is far more healthful and natural for their species. They can also often substantially cut their food costs by growing food in their own gardens, ideally using organic farming methods.

Some are also inspired by the Biblical quote from Genesis 1:29 in which God told the humans in the Garden of Eden: "I give you every seed-bearing plant on the face of the whole earth and every tree that has fruit with seed in it. They will be yours for food. " (New International Version)

Although not absolutely necessary, most committed raw vegans will also develop expertise in sprouting various types of seeds, legumes and grains in order to activate them and increase their mass, nutritive value and edibility. With time, they can also learn to replicate just about any cooked food dish with raw vegan substitutes that can be processed from fresh fruits and vegetables, soaked nuts and seeds, and sprouted grains and legumes.

Some elements of these raw dishes might require dehydration at temperatures below 117 degrees Fahrenheit to achieve certain desirable textures. Examples include flax crackers and various Essene bread recipes, as well as the nut loaf, raw pizza and falafel recipes provided in the recipe section of this book that were very popular entrées at my raw vegan restaurant. The nut loaf was also generally served topped with sun dried tomato ketchup and with date mustard and cauliflower garlic "mashed potatoes" on the side, which you can find recipes for in Part II of this book.

Live and Let Live

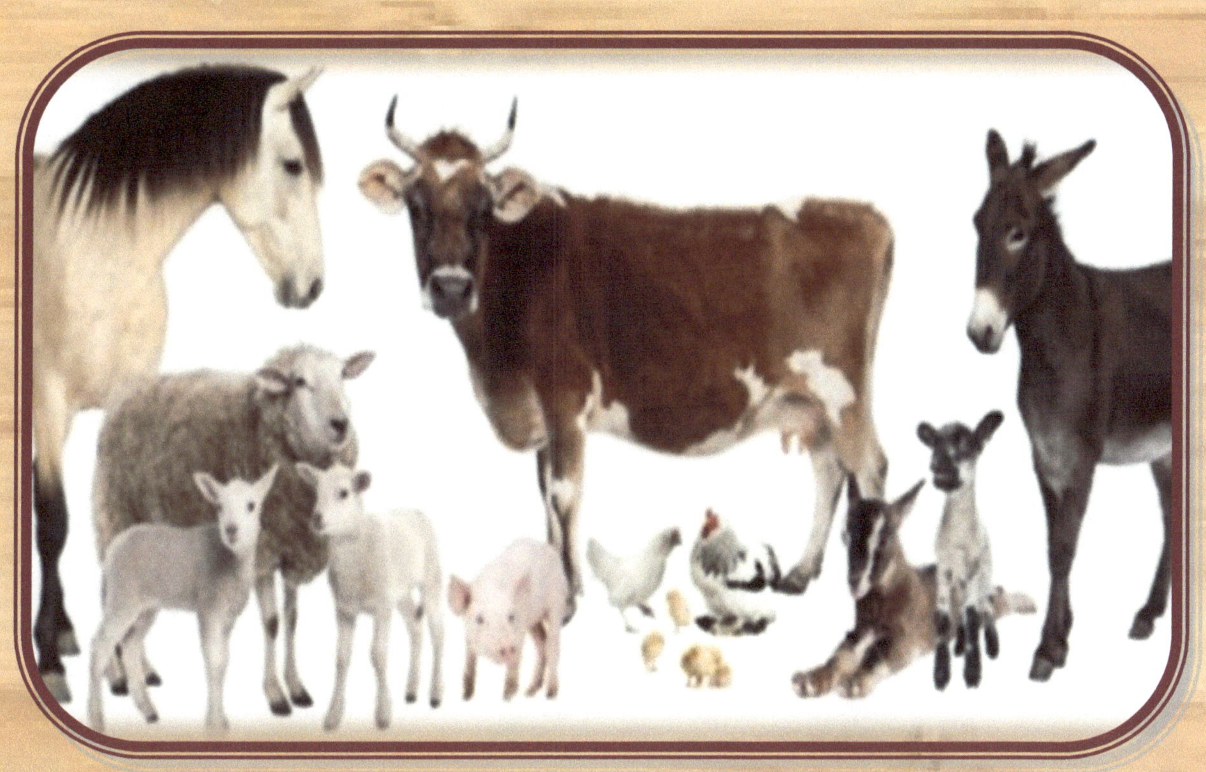

Perhaps the highest and best reason to maintain a vegan diet is that it is free of products that contribute unnecessarily to animal cruelty and suffering. The fact that farmed animals suffer when mistreated, tightly confined and violently killed — as they are in virtually all intensive animal agricultural facilities and slaughterhouses — is scientifically indisputable at this point.

All humans who consistently abstain from animal products can generally achieve a clearer conscience because they are not unnecessarily contributing to the suffering, exploitation and involuntary death of animals by buying and eating their flesh or other products. Abstaining from supporting this violence and animal abuse will also greatly reduce your karmic burden.

Furthermore, returning to your natural diet consisting of whole, plant-derived foods will typically allow you to live a healthier lifestyle and enjoy a longer life. Going a step further to consume a raw vegan diet has numerous additional health benefits too, and when all is said and done, nothing is healthier than a clear conscience and consuming a natural diet for your species.

Basically, following a raw vegan diet allows virtually anyone to enjoy a healthier life, and as you will soon discover, you can dine on delicious and creative plant-based dishes free of the unnecessary guilt that harming others can induce in a person who truly cares about animals. Raw vegans really do enjoy a win-win situation as their diet affirms both their life and that of others!

Become a Temple
Not a Graveyard

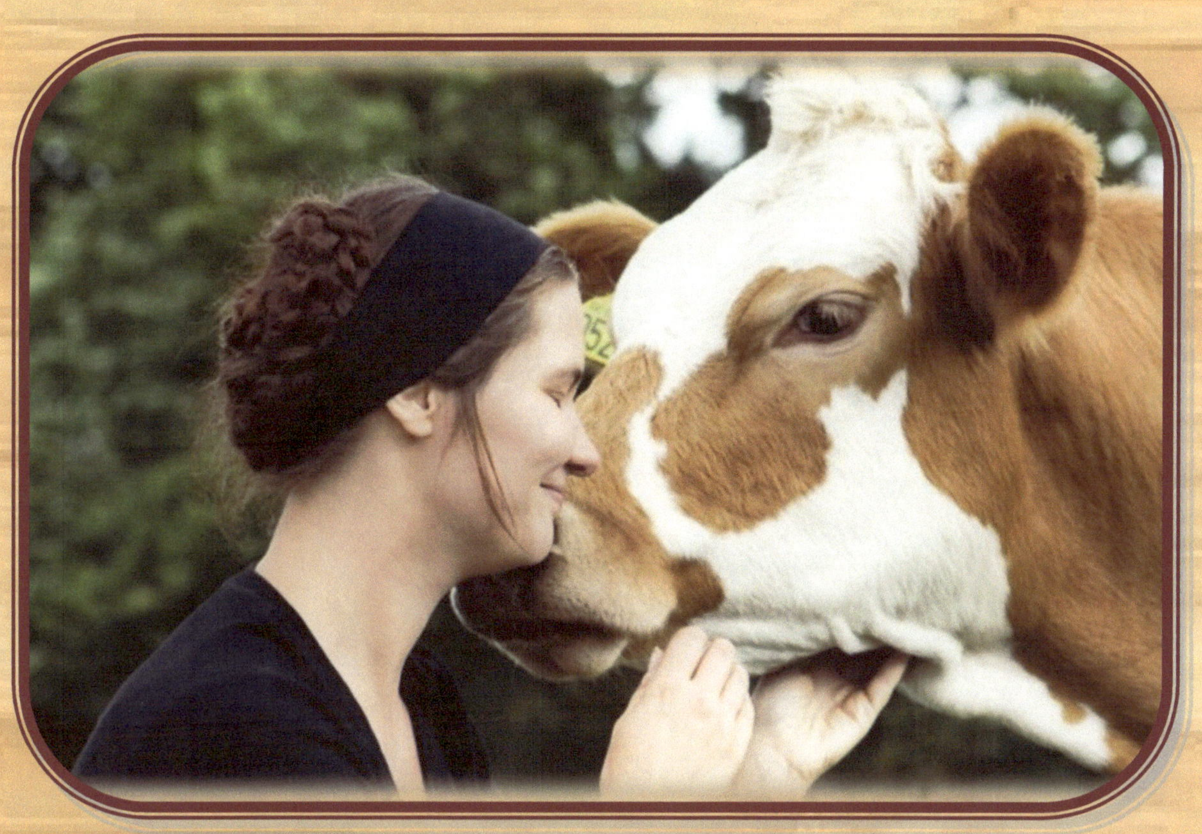

Once you have resolved to let your body become a temple for your soul instead of a graveyard for your fellow creatures by embracing the vegan lifestyle, you can expect some delightful results from your new natural, healthful and highly ethical diet.

As a vegan, prepare to allow your heart to open to all sentient beings as they no longer have anything to fear from you. Furthermore, by enjoying a raw, whole foods, plant-based diet, you will wisely be consuming natural foods that are just right for your species.

Not only will you clear your conscience as a raw vegan, but you will clear up your complexion and your digestive and circulatory systems at the same time.

In many cases, chronic diseases like diabetes, cancer, heart disease and excess weight will also melt away like snow in the sun, and your energy levels will be remarkable as a raw vegan.

Even the aging process should slow down as you consume far more vitalizing raw plant foods full of biophotons and valuable micronutrients that have been shown to help extend your lifespan and make you look younger.

Your mood should also improve, and many people find the raw diet helps them make their way out of depression and towards a lasting sense of happiness and contentment.

Overall, you can hardly do a better thing for your health, your mood, your planet and your fellow creatures than go raw vegan today!